# METABOLIC REBOOT

## FROM CRISIS TO CURE WITH THE POWER OF FOOD

JAMES AND CRYSTAL BASS

Metabolic Reboot

**From Crisis to Cure with The Power of Food**

By

**James and Crystal Bass**

Published by Clarice Jefferies Publishing

Contact info: cjpublishing@yahoo.com

Copyright © 2025 James Bass

All rights reserved

For permissions, contact:

cjpublishing@yahoo.com

Printed in the United States of America on responsibly sourced paper

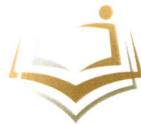

CLARICE JEFFERIES

## Disclaimer

The information in this book is meant to be educational and provide a foundation for understanding health-related topics, but it's not a substitute for professional medical advice. If you have questions or concerns about a medical condition, always consult your doctor or another qualified healthcare professional. Never ignore or delay seeking professional advice because of something you've read in this book.

This book is not intended to diagnose, treat, prescribe, or cure any illness. We're simply sharing our personal experiences and the lessons we've learned along the way. Keep in mind that science and nutritional information are always evolving, so the details about foods and supplements mentioned here might have changed. Be sure to do your own research and stay informed as you navigate your health journey!

### 1 Corinthians 10:31 (NIV):
*"So whether you eat or drink or whatever you do,
do it all for the glory of God."*

### Genesis 1:29 (NIV):
*"Then God said, 'I give you every seedbearing plant on the
face of the whole earth and every tree that has fruit with seed
in it. They will be yours for food.'"*

### Ezekiel 4:9 (NIV):
*"Take wheat and barley, beans and lentils, millet and spelt;
put them in a storage jar and use them to make
bread for yourself."*

*"The food you eat can be either the safest and most powerful
form of medicine, or the slowest form of poison."*
### - Ann Wigmore

*"Let food be thy medicine and medicine be thy food. I will
apply dietetic measures for the benefit of the sick according to
my ability and judgement; I will keep them from harm and
injustice. I will neither give a deadly drug to anybody who
asked for it, nor will I make a suggestion to this effect. "*
### - Hippocrates

*"The doctor of the future will no longer treat the human
frame with drugs, but rather will cure and prevent disease
with nutrition."*
### - Thomas Edison

# TABLE OF CONTENTS

# THE DIAGNOSIS

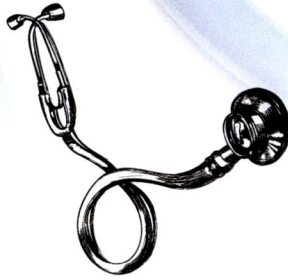

In the early months of 2012, Crystal began to experience persistent, unexplained discomfort. What initially seemed like a minor nuisance—a subtle ache in her bones that we attributed to the natural toll of time or simple fatigue—soon evolved into something far more troubling. As the weeks turned into months, her pain intensified, and with it came a growing sense of unease. It became increasingly clear that this was not a transient ailment but a sign of something more insidious.

Medical professionals approached her case with diligence and compassion. They conducted a thorough review of her history and ordered a comprehensive panel of diagnostic tests. Blood was drawn, and with each passing day of waiting, anxiety thickened the air around us. The uncertainty was excruciating—each moment suspended between fear and fragile hope, the unknown steadily eroding our peace of mind.

When the call finally came, it confirmed our worst suspicions. Crystal's **alkaline phosphatase** levels were significantly elevated—a biomarker that signaled a possible underlying bone disorder. It was a sobering revelation that felt like a gathering storm had suddenly broken, its full force crashing down upon us.

Doctors recommended a CT scan of her bones and skull to gain further clarity. That day was marked by a tense, unspoken dread. The scanning process was brief, but the emotional weight was immense. Each tick of the clock seemed stretched, the minutes dragging as we braced ourselves for what the images might reveal.

The results were devastating. The scans confirmed the presence of both **arthritis** and **Paget's Disease of The Bone**—a chronic, progressive condition that would remain with Crystal for the rest of her life. Hearing the diagnosis was like having the ground pulled from beneath us. The magnitude of the news landed with crushing finality, burying our hopes beneath the harsh reality of what lay ahead.

The physician explained the nature of the disease with solemn clarity: it was irreversible, unpredictable, and would gradually reshape the course of Crystal's life. I watched her face as the words sank in.

Her eyes welled with a complexity of emotion—fear, sorrow, disbelief. At that moment, time seemed to pause, the world around us dimming under the weight of what we had just been told.

And yet, amid that sorrow, a quiet resolve emerged. I reached for her hand, silently vowing we would confront this new reality together. Our bond—strengthened over years of shared joys and struggles—would now be our foundation. We would meet this trial not in isolation but side by side.

That day marked a profound turning point in our lives. The road ahead was uncertain and difficult, but our love remained unchanged—anchoring us against the rising tide. As the sun dipped below the horizon, we found solace in each other, determined to face whatever came next with courage, compassion, and unwavering unity.

# ALKALINE PHOSPHATASE

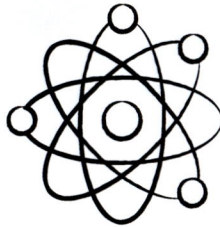

**A**lkaline phosphatase (ALP) is an essential enzyme found throughout the body, most prominently in the liver, bones, kidneys, intestines, and—during pregnancy—in the placenta. It plays a crucial role in numerous physiological processes, including bone formation, liver function, and nutrient metabolism. While exact reference ranges may vary slightly from one laboratory to another, the normal range of ALP typically falls between 25 and 100 international units per liter (U/L).

Crystal's levels came back at **532.**

The number hit like a thunderclap—startling, ominous, and impossible to ignore. It was far beyond what would be expected, even under strained physical conditions. In the sterile language of the lab report, it was just a number. But to us, it was a signal—a red flag waving urgently, alerting us to the gravity of what might be unfolding within her body.

To understand the emotional weight of that number, one must understand the role ALP plays. It is not just a routine figure on a blood panel; it is a window into the quiet, intricate workings of the human body. In the bones, ALP facilitates growth and repair, enabling the deposition of minerals like calcium and phosphate that keep the skeletal structure strong.

In the liver, it contributes to the transport and processing of nutrients, and its elevation can signal liver stress or disease. During pregnancy, levels naturally rise to support fetal development, a biological adaptation that underscores how responsive this enzyme is to the body's demands. But Crystal wasn't pregnant. And her liver showed no signs of distress.

The implication was chilling. Elevated ALP, especially when not tied to liver dysfunction, often points to bone turnover—abnormally increased activity in bone formation or breakdown. For Crystal, that likely meant a metabolic bone disorder, the kind that wears away at the very foundation of the body.

We didn't yet have a name for what was happening, but that number—532—hung in the air like a shadow. It turned our concern into fear. It took an ambiguous pain and made it tangible, clinical, and measurable. It marked the beginning of a new chapter in which medical terms would become daily vocabulary, and our emotional endurance would be tested in ways we had never imagined.

This wasn't just data. It was the first true sign that Crystal's pain was not a phantom, not a passing discomfort. It was the body's quiet cry for help, finally heard through the language of enzymes and numbers.

# PAGET'S DISEASE OF THE BONE

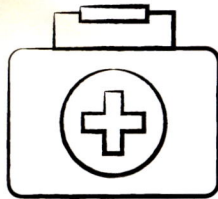

P aget's disease of the bone is a chronic and progressive disorder that disrupts the body's natural bone remodeling process—a delicate balance of breakdown and renewal that keeps the skeletal system strong and structurally sound. In individuals with this condition, that process becomes chaotic and inefficient. The bones are broken down too quickly and rebuilt in a disorganized fashion, resulting in structures that are enlarged, weakened, and often painfully deformed.

For Crystal, the diagnosis of Paget's disease was more than just a clinical label—it was a seismic shift in her life. It marked the moment when vague pain transformed into a lifelong condition, and uncertainty crystallized into an unrelenting reality.

One of the most telling biochemical indicators of Paget's disease is the elevated presence of alkaline phosphatase (ALP) in the blood. This enzyme, typically found in the liver and bones, plays a central role in bone metabolism. In healthy adults, ALP levels usually range between 25 and 100 international units per liter (U/L). Crystal's level was 532—a number so far outside the normal parameters that it offered immediate and unsettling clarity.

This elevation wasn't incidental. It was the direct result of excessive bone turnover—the hallmark of Paget's disease. In the disorder, the cells responsible for bone remodeling—osteoclasts that break down bone and osteoblasts that rebuild it—become hyperactive. The result is a frenzied construction site within the skeleton, where the bone is being broken down and rebuilt at an accelerated pace but with poor architectural integrity. As this activity intensifies, ALP is released into the bloodstream in elevated quantities, serving as a biochemical flare that something is terribly wrong.

In Crystal's case, this elevated enzyme level, combined with her escalating pain and the radiological evidence of bone irregularities, formed the unmistakable fingerprint of Paget's disease.

The diagnosis was not arrived at lightly—it was confirmed through careful correlation of symptoms, blood chemistry, and imaging studies. But once confirmed, it carried immense emotional weight.

To be told that one's bones—the very framework of the body— is gradually weakening and deforming is to confront a profound and existential vulnerability. For Crystal, the realization was devastating. The disease would not only cause chronic discomfort and fatigue;

it would also become a persistent, invisible burden. There would be medications to manage the symptoms, frequent monitoring, and a constant awareness of fragility in the very structure of her body.

Yet even amid the grief, there was clarity. We now had a name for what had been silently eroding her strength. The numbers and scans told a story we could finally begin to understand. And with understanding came the first step toward action, however daunting that path would be.

Paget's disease, with all its clinical terminology and measurable metrics, is still, at its core, a profoundly human affliction—one that reshapes not only the bones of the body but the contours of everyday life. Crystal's journey was beginning, and though the road ahead was uncertain, we faced it with the strength that comes from knowledge, love, and a shared determination to endure.

# OUR SKELETAL SYSTEM'S REGENERATION PROCESS

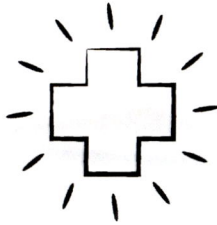

**T**he human skeletal system is one of the body's most extraordinary and resilient structures. Often thought of as static, it is a living, breathing framework that is constantly renewing itself. This continuous regeneration is vital for maintaining strength and structural integrity, adapting to the evolving physical demands of life, and healing from injury.

At the core of this renewal is a process known as **bone remodeling**—a sophisticated and lifelong biological cycle in which old bone tissue is systematically broken down and replaced with new. Two specialized types of cells orchestrate this complex task:

- **Osteoclasts** act as the system's demolition crew. These cells break down aged or damaged bone, creating space for fresh growth.

- **Osteoblasts** are the builders, depositing minerals such as calcium and phosphate to form new bone and restore the structural integrity that may have been lost through age, injury, or stress.

This interplay between destruction and renewal is more than mere maintenance—it is the silent work that keeps us upright, mobile, and protected throughout our lives. Bone remodeling supports three essential functions:

1. **Preservation of strength**: It ensures that bones remain resilient under the constant pressures of daily life—bearing weight, supporting motion, and protecting vital organs.

2. **Adaptation to physical demands**: The skeleton responds to how we use our bodies. For instance, someone beginning a regimen of weight-bearing exercise may stimulate their bones to become denser and more robust in response.

3. **Repair after injury**: When fractures or micro-damage occur, this process steps in to rebuild, often stronger than before.

The entire human skeleton is gradually replaced approximately every **ten years**. This process isn't uniform—certain bones, like those in the legs and arms, undergo more frequent remodeling due to their active role in movement and weight-bearing. Others, like the bones of the skull, remodel more slowly.

Over a typical lifespan, the entire skeletal system may be renewed **10 to 15 times**, depending on a range of factors, including genetics, hormonal health, nutrition, and physical activity. This quiet rhythm of breakdown and rebuilding often goes unnoticed—until something interrupts it.

In Crystal's case, this fundamental process had begun to falter. What should have been a seamless renewal cycle had turned chaotic and erratic. The balance between osteoclasts and osteoblasts had been lost with the onset of Paget's disease. Her bones, once strong and efficient in their renewal, were now remodeling at an accelerated and disorganized pace—growing larger, weaker, and increasingly prone to pain and deformity.

This insight was more than a physiological fact; it became the emotional linchpin of her diagnosis. To know that the very foundation of her body was betraying her, not in a sudden collapse but in gradual, uncontrollable disarray, was a grief that went beyond physical suffering. Her skeleton—the unseen support of every step, gesture, and breath—had become unreliable. And with that realization came a deeper emotional weight: the body she had always trusted was no longer working in her favor.

Understanding the science behind bone remodeling helped us frame the scope of her condition. But it did not soften the emotional blow. The knowledge carried clarity, yes—but also a sobering permanence. Her bones would not heal in the way other injuries might. They would need to be monitored, managed, and cared for constantly for the rest of her life.

And so, while the science offered answers, it also marked the beginning of an emotional journey—mourning what had been lost and learning to live with a new, unpredictable reality.

# OUR BODIES SYSTEMS

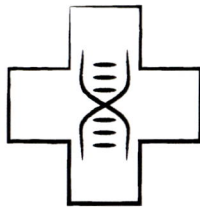

T he human body is a profoundly intricate and resilient biological system composed of interconnected networks that work harmoniously to sustain life. From a young age, we are introduced to the concept of body systems in school, often beginning with five fundamental ones. As our understanding deepens, so does our appreciation for the breadth of physiological processes that occur silently and tirelessly within us every second of every day.

**Foundational Body Systems and Their Vital Roles:**

**Circulatory (Cardiovascular) System**

Often referred to as the body's transportation highway, the circulatory system ensures the delivery of oxygen, nutrients, hormones, and immune cells to every tissue while removing metabolic waste. Comprising of the heart, blood vessels, and blood, this system is central to our survival—its rhythmic pulse is a constant reminder of life itself.

### Respiratory System

Breath by breath, the respiratory system connects our internal world with the environment. Oxygen is drawn in through the nose, trachea, bronchi, lungs, and diaphragm, and carbon dioxide is expelled. When compromised, even the simple act of breathing becomes a desperate struggle—a sobering reminder of this system's critical function.

### Nervous System

As the body's command center, the nervous system governs thought, sensation, movement, and reflexes. It bridges the mind and body through a vast network of neurons, the brain, spinal cord, and peripheral nerves. It is the essence of who we are—coordinating the electrical symphony that animates our being.

### Digestive System

More than a mechanism for processing food, the digestive system converts sustenance into life-sustaining energy. Beginning in the mouth and ending in the intestines, it fuels every organ. When disrupted, it affects energy levels, immunity, and mood, making us keenly aware of its foundational role in daily wellness.

### Musculoskeletal System

The musculoskeletal system forms the physical foundation of our bodies—providing structure, movement, and protection. Bones, muscles, ligaments, and tendons work in unison to allow motion and bear the weight of life. When compromised, the loss of independence or mobility can deeply affect one's sense of identity and autonomy.

## Expanded Systems: The Full Spectrum of Human Physiology

As we grow in understanding, we come to recognize additional systems that are just as essential:

- **Endocrine System:** Regulates metabolism, growth, reproduction, and mood through a precise cascade of hormones released by glands like the thyroid, pancreas, and adrenal glands.

- **Immune System:** Defends the body against pathogens. Its complexity is matched only by its vigilance—silently scanning, identifying, and neutralizing threats.

- **Integumentary System:** The skin, hair, and nails form a protective barrier while also regulating temperature and sensory perception.

- **Reproductive System:** Ensures the continuation of the species through the production of gametes and hormonal cycles, and in females, nurtures new life.

- **Urinary System:** Filters blood, removes waste, and maintains electrolyte balance through the production and excretion of urine.

- **Lymphatic System:** Works with the immune system to maintain fluid balance and facilitate immune surveillance via lymphatic vessels and nodes.

- **Sensory System:** Comprising the eyes, ears, skin, tongue, and nose, it interprets the external world—allowing us to see beauty, hear music, taste food, and feel touch.

- **Endocannabinoid System:** A lesser known but vital modulator of sleep, pain, appetite, and emotional balance.

- **Excretory System:** A collective of organs involved in eliminating waste, ensuring internal cleanliness, and chemical homeostasis.

**Nutrition: The Lifeblood of Systemic Health**

Each body system depends on a unique blend of minerals, vitamins, and nutrients. Deficiencies impair function and can deeply disrupt one's physical and emotional well-being. Below is an overview of the critical nutrients for each system, the fruits and vegetables that supply them, and the potential consequences of deficiency:

### 1. Skeletal System

- **Key Nutrients:** Calcium, Vitamin D, Magnesium, Phosphorus, Vitamin K

- **Deficiency Risks:** Osteoporosis, fractures, stunted growth

- **Helpful Foods:** Kale, spinach, broccoli, oranges, kiwi

### 2. Muscular System

- **Key Nutrients:** Protein, Calcium, Potassium, Vitamin D, B-complex

- **Deficiency Risks:** Muscle weakness, spasms, poor coordination

- **Helpful Foods:** Bananas, sweet potatoes, lentils, avocados

## 3. Circulatory System

- **Key Nutrients:** Iron, B vitamins, Vitamin C, Potassium
- **Deficiency Risks:** Anemia, fatigue, poor circulation
- **Helpful Foods:** Berries, citrus fruits, spinach, beets

## 4. Respiratory System

- **Key Nutrients:** Vitamin D, Magnesium, Vitamin A, Omega-3s
- **Deficiency Risks:** Respiratory infections, reduced lung function
- **Helpful Foods:** Carrots, pumpkin, broccoli, oranges

## 5. Nervous System

- **Key Nutrients:** B12, Folate, Magnesium, Omega-3s
- **Deficiency Risks:** Cognitive decline, nerve damage
- **Helpful Foods:** Avocados, walnuts, blueberries, almonds

## 6. Digestive System

- **Key Nutrients:** Fiber, B-complex, Magnesium
- **Deficiency Risks:** Constipation, gut inflammation
- **Helpful Foods:** Apples, kiwi, bananas, ginger

## 7. Endocrine System

- **Key Nutrients:** Iodine, Zinc, Selenium, Vitamin D
- **Deficiency Risks:** Hormonal imbalance, thyroid disorders
- **Helpful Foods:** Seaweed, legumes, dairy, leafy greens

### 8. Immune System

- **Key Nutrients:** Vitamin C, Zinc, Selenium, Vitamin D
- **Deficiency Risks:** Frequent illness, slow healing
- **Helpful Foods:** Garlic, berries, bell peppers, spinach

### 9. Reproductive System

- **Key Nutrients:** Folic acid, Iron, Vitamin E
- **Deficiency Risks:** Fertility issues, neural tube defects
- **Helpful Foods:** Dark leafy greens, nuts, berries, avocados

### 10. Urinary System

- **Key Nutrients:** Water, Potassium, Magnesium
- **Deficiency Risks:** Kidney stones, fluid imbalance
- **Helpful Foods:** Watermelon, tomatoes, citrus fruits

### 11. Integumentary System

- **Key Nutrients:** Vitamin A, E, C, Biotin, Zinc
- **Deficiency Risks:** Skin issues, hair loss, slow healing
- **Helpful Foods:** Carrots, sweet potatoes, berries, citrus

Ensure a balanced diet by incorporating a variety of fruits and vegetables into your meals to meet the needs of all body systems. Always consult a healthcare professional for personalized dietary advice.

# ORGANIC FOODS WE EAT & SUPPLEMENTS WE TAKE

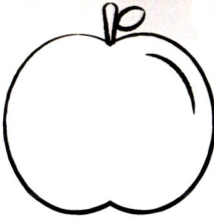

In today's increasingly health-conscious world, organic foods and herbal supplements have gained recognition for their nutrient-dense profiles and therapeutic potential. These natural remedies have long been used in traditional medicine and are now seeing a resurgence due to growing interest in holistic health. Below is a detailed exploration of the organic supplements and foods we eat, their bioactive constituents, and the science-backed health benefits they may offer.

## 1. Elderberry Syrup and Echinacea

## Immune-Enhancing Herbal Remedies

**Elderberry (Sambucus nigra)** and **Echinacea** are two of the most commonly used botanicals for immune support, especially during the cold and flu season.

### Elderberry Syrup

### Key Constituents:

- **Flavonoids (quercetin, rutin, kaempferol):** Antioxidants that protect cells from oxidative damage.

- **Anthocyanins:** Pigments with potent antioxidant and anti-inflammatory properties.

- **Vitamins A, B, and C, and minerals like iron, copper, and potassium.**

### Health Benefits:

- **Immune Support:** Boosts immune response during viral infections.

- **Antiviral Potential:** May inhibit the replication of flu viruses.

- **Anti-inflammatory:** Reduces inflammation and related symptoms.

- **Antioxidant Protection:** Fights oxidative stress, supporting cellular health.

**Echinacea**

**Key Constituents:**

- **Alkamides:** Stimulate immune function.

- **Polyphenols and Polysaccharides:** Offer antioxidant and immune-enhancing properties.

**Health Benefits:**

- **Cold and Flu Relief:** May reduce the duration and severity of respiratory infections.

- **Wound Healing:** Used topically for minor cuts and skin conditions.

- **Anti-inflammatory Effects:** Helps manage inflammatory conditions like arthritis.

**Note:** While both remedies have promising effects, users should consult a healthcare professional for guidance, particularly those with chronic conditions or those who are pregnant.

## 2. Maca Root and Ashwagandha

### Adaptogenic Herbs for Stress, Energy, and Hormonal Balance

**Maca Root (Lepidium meyenii)** and **Ashwagandha (Withania somnifera)** are revered in traditional Peruvian and Ayurvedic medicine, respectively, for their ability to help the body cope with stress and maintain equilibrium.

### Maca Root

### Key Constituents:

- **Macamides & Macaenes:** Linked to increased stamina and libido.

- **Glucosinolates and Alkaloids:** May offer antioxidant and neurological benefits.

- **Vitamins (B-complex, C) and Minerals (iron, copper, potassium).**

### Health Benefits:

- **Hormonal Balance:** Especially beneficial for menopausal symptoms and fertility.

- **Energy and Endurance:** Used by athletes and those with chronic fatigue.

- **Cognitive Enhancement:** May support learning and memory functions.

**Ashwagandha**

**Key Constituents:**

- **Withanolides and Alkaloids:** Contribute to anti-stress and immune-boosting effects.

- **Saponins:** Support inflammation control and immune modulation.

**Health Benefits:**

- **Stress Reduction:** Lowers cortisol levels and improves resilience.

- **Sleep Support:** Enhances sleep quality.

- **Cognitive and Immune Function:** Improves mental clarity and strengthens immunity.

**Caution:** Individuals with thyroid conditions or those on medication should use it under medical supervision.

## 3. Black Cumin Seed Oil (Nigella sativa)

### A Versatile Oil for Immune, Metabolic, and Digestive Health

**Key Constituents:**

- **Thymoquinone, Thymohydroquinone, and Thymol:** Provide antimicrobial, antioxidant, and anti-inflammatory effects.

- **Alpha-hederin, Essential Fatty Acids:** Contribute to cellular health and immune support.

**Health Benefits:**

- **Immune System Enhancement:** Boosts natural defenses.

- **Anti-inflammatory and Antioxidant Effects:** Supports management of asthma, arthritis, and oxidative stress.

- **Digestive and Cardiovascular Health:** Promotes gastrointestinal function and may improve lipid profiles.

- **Antimicrobial Properties:** Useful against bacterial and fungal infections.

Black cumin seed oil is potent and should be used in controlled amounts under professional guidance.

## 4. Chlorella and Spirulina

## Superfoods from Algae for Detoxification and Cellular Health

Both **Chlorella** and **Spirulina** are nutrient-rich algae with substantial health benefits.

### Chlorella

### Key Constituents:

- **Chlorophyll, Beta-glucans, Nucleic Acids:** Aid in detoxification and immunity.
- **Vitamins C, E, and B-complex; Minerals like iron and calcium.**

### Health Benefits:

- **Detoxification:** Binds heavy metals and supports liver detox.
- **Immune Boost:** Stimulates white blood cell production.
- **Digestive Support:** High in fiber and enzymes.
- **Antioxidant Defense:** Protects against cellular damage.

### Spirulina

### Key Constituents:

- **Phycocyanin, GLA (Gamma-linolenic acid):** Anti-inflammatory and antioxidant agents.
- **Vitamins B1, B2, K, and Minerals like magnesium and iron.**

**Health Benefits:**

- **Complete Protein Source:** Ideal for plant-based diets.

- **Reduces Inflammation:** Beneficial in chronic conditions.

- **Potential Anti-cancer Properties:** Research suggests inhibition of cancer cell growth.

These superfoods are excellent dietary additions but should be introduced gradually and with expert advice for those with sensitivities.

## 5. Alfalfa and Moringa Powders

**Nutritional Powerhouses for Energy, Immunity, and Heart Health**

**Alfalfa**

**Key Constituents:**

- **Vitamins A, C, E, and K; Minerals like calcium, iron, and magnesium.**
- **Chlorophyll and Fiber:** Aid detoxification and digestion.

**Health Benefits:**

- **Nutrient Supplementation:** Helps address dietary deficiencies.
- **Cholesterol and Blood Sugar Control:** Potential in managing metabolic conditions.
- **Antioxidant Protection and Bone Support.**

**Moringa**

**Key Constituents:**

- **Vitamins A, B6, C, D, and E; Protein and Iron.**
- **Flavonoids and Polyphenols:** Offer strong antioxidant support.

**Health Benefits:**

- **Energy and Immune Function:** Supports metabolic and immune responses.
- **Anti-inflammatory and Anti-diabetic Effects:** May help manage chronic conditions.
- **Supports Heart and Digestive Health.**

## 6. Sprouted Pumpkin Seeds and Brazil Nuts

### Nutrient-Dense Snacks for Vital Health Functions

### Sprouted Pumpkin Seeds

**Key Nutrients:**

- **Omega-3 and Omega-6, Zinc, Magnesium, Protein, Fiber.**

**Health Benefits:**

- **Immune and Cardiovascular Support:** Thanks to high zinc and healthy fat content.

- **Digestive and Muscle Health:** Fiber and protein contribute to regularity and repair.

### Brazil Nuts

**Key Nutrients:**

- **Selenium, Magnesium, Copper, Healthy Fats, Protein.**

**Health Benefits:**

- **Thyroid Function:** Selenium supports hormone production.

- **Mood and Cognitive Support:** Selenium is linked to reduced depression and improved brain function.

- **Bone and Antioxidant Health:** Combats oxidative stress and supports bone density.

Brazil nuts are incredibly selenium-rich—limit intake to avoid overconsumption.

## 7. Broccoli and Kale

## Cruciferous Vegetables for Disease Prevention and Detox

These vegetables are nutrient-dense staples known for their cancer-preventive properties and detoxifying effects.

### Broccoli

### Nutritional Highlights:

- **Vitamins C, K, A; Sulforaphane, Fiber, Potassium.**

### Health Benefits:

- **Supports Immune and Bone Health:** Via vitamins K and C.

- **Detoxification and Anti-cancer Properties:** Due to sulforaphane and glucosinolates.

### Kale

### Nutritional Highlights:

- **Vitamins A, K, and C; Lutein, Zeaxanthin, Calcium, Iron.**

### Health Benefits:

- **Eye Health:** High in vision-supportive carotenoids.

- **Antioxidant Support:** Reduces chronic disease risk.

- **Liver Detoxification and Heart Health.**

## Bell Peppers: A Spectrum of Color, A Wealth of Health

Bell peppers—red, green, and yellow—are far more than culinary accents. Each vibrant color signals a distinct profile of vitamins, antioxidants, and phytochemicals. Beyond their crisp sweetness lies a potent source of preventive health.

### Red Bell Peppers

- **Vitamin C**: Extremely rich in vitamin C, red peppers support immune strength, collagen production, and iron absorption.

- **Beta-Carotene (Vitamin A precursor)**: Promotes visual acuity, skin repair, and immune function.

- **Vitamin B6 & Folate**: Essential for neurological development, mood regulation, and red blood cell production.

- **Lycopene**: A potent antioxidant associated with lowered risk of prostate cancer and cardiovascular disease.

- **Antioxidants**: Reduce systemic inflammation and oxidative stress—a contributor to aging and chronic illness.

### Green Bell Peppers

- **Vitamin K**: Crucial for bone density and effective blood clotting.

- **Dietary Fiber**: Enhances digestion, stabilizes blood sugar, and contributes to satiety.

- **Moderate Vitamin C & Beta-Carotene**: Still valuable for immune support and cell protection.

### Yellow Bell Peppers

- **Vitamin C & A**: Support immunity and skin health.

- **Folate (Vitamin B9)**: Important for DNA synthesis, especially during pregnancy.

- **Carotenoids (Lutein, Zeaxanthin)**: Protect the eyes from age-related macular degeneration and oxidative damage.

### Cumulative Benefits of Bell Peppers

- **Immune Support**: High vitamin C and A content bolster the body's natural defenses.

- **Eye Health**: Beta-carotene, lutein, and zeaxanthin shield vision from decline.

- **Heart Protection**: Antioxidants and fiber help regulate cholesterol and support vascular health.

- **Digestive Balance**: Natural fiber promotes gut regularity and a healthy microbiome.

*Incorporating bell peppers of all colors into the diet offers a full spectrum of preventive nutrients. Their vibrant presence on the plate is a reminder of nature's design to heal and sustain us.*

**Watermelon and Kiwi**

**Hydration, Nourishment, and Cellular Defense**

Nature's fruits often come as sweet reminders of life's simplest joys. Watermelon and kiwi stand out for their flavor and profound ability to nourish and protect the human body on a cellular level.

**Watermelon**

- **Hydration Powerhouse**: Composed of over 90% water, it is essential in regulating body temperature, supporting organ function, and reducing fatigue.

- **Vitamin A & C**: Support immune responses, vision, and tissue repair.

- **Lycopene**: Fights oxidative stress, supports heart and prostate health, and protects skin from UV damage.

- **Citrulline**: Converts to arginine, a compound that improves circulation and may enhance exercise performance.

- **Minerals (Potassium, Magnesium)**: Help maintain normal blood pressure and support muscle and nerve function.

*Watermelon's Role in Well-being*

- **Cardiovascular Support**: Lycopene and potassium work together to reduce hypertension risk.

- **Post-Workout Recovery**: Citrulline aids in reducing muscle soreness and promoting recovery.

- **Skin Health**: A mix of hydration and antioxidants slows premature aging and improves skin tone.

## Kiwi

- **Exceptionally High Vitamin C**: One kiwi exceeds the daily recommended intake, reinforcing immunity and skin integrity.

- **Dietary Fiber**: Promotes digestive health, regulates glucose absorption, and nourishes gut bacteria.

- **Antioxidants (Flavonoids & Carotenoids)**: Combat free radical damage and reduce inflammation.

- **Minerals (Potassium, Calcium)**: Aid in blood pressure regulation and bone mineralization.

- **Folate & Vitamin K**: Crucial for fetal development and bone integrity.

### *Kiwi's Holistic Impact*

- **Immune Defense**: High vitamin C helps prevent colds and speeds recovery.

- **Digestive Harmony**: Natural enzymes and fibers ease digestion.

- **Heart and Bone Strength**: Potassium and vitamin K lower stroke risk and enhance bone density.

*Fruits like watermelon and kiwi are nature's subtle medicine—offering not just flavor but deeply restorative, hydrating, and healing qualities that support the rhythm of life itself.*

## Wild-Caught Alaskan Salmon and Sardines: Oceanic Superfoods for Modern Wellness

From the cold, pristine waters of the ocean come two of the most nutrient-dense foods known to science. Wild-caught Alaskan salmon and sardines offer a sustainable, accessible, and profound way to fortify the human body—especially in a world where inflammation, heart disease, and neurodegenerative conditions are on the rise.

### Wild-Caught Alaskan Salmon

- **Omega-3 Fatty Acids (EPA & DHA)**: Support heart rhythm, reduce inflammation, and form the building blocks of the brain.

- **Complete Protein**: Assists in tissue repair, immune regulation, and hormonal balance.

- **Vitamin D**: Essential for bone metabolism, immune vigilance, and mental well-being.

- **B-Vitamins (B12, Niacin, B6)**: Fuel energy metabolism and protect cognitive function.

- **Selenium & Phosphorus**: Shield the body from oxidative stress and strengthen skeletal integrity.

- **Astaxanthin**: Gives salmon its pink hue and protects skin and brain cells from oxidative aging.

-

### Salmon's Transformative Health Benefits

- **Cardiovascular Integrity**: Omega-3s reduce triglycerides and promote flexible blood vessels.

- **Cognitive Longevity**: DHA supports memory, mood, and neural resilience.

- **Inflammation Control**: Supports joint health and may ease autoimmune flare-ups.

- **Eye Protection**: Helps prevent macular degeneration and dry eye syndrome.

### Sardines

- **Rich in EPA & DHA Omega-3s**: Deliver heart and brain benefits similar to salmon, often with lower environmental toxins.

- **Calcium & Vitamin D**: Promote bone density, especially valuable for those at risk of osteoporosis.

- **Vitamin B12**: Vital for neurological stability and energy production.

- **Selenium & Phosphorus**: Antioxidant defense and cell repair.

- **Protein**: Sustainably sourced and easily digestible.

### Sardines' Health Contributions

- **Heart Protection**: Omega-3s support vascular health and reduce systemic inflammation.

- **Bone Preservation**: High calcium content is critical in aging populations.

- **Mental Health:** B12 and omega-3s support mood and reduce the risk of cognitive decline.

*Eating seafood like wild salmon and sardines isn't just about personal nutrition—it's a deeply meaningful choice rooted in sustainability, ancestral wisdom, and the protection of life itself.*

### Cacao: A Mood-Boosting Superfood

Cacao, the core ingredient of chocolate, is derived from the **Theobroma cacao** tree and is cherished for both its rich, deep flavor and impressive health benefits. Beyond its taste, cacao carries an emotional essence, often associated with comfort, indulgence, and happiness.

### 1. Antioxidants and Cardiovascular Health:

- Cacao is abundant in flavonoids, particularly flavanols, which are potent antioxidants that help protect cells from oxidative damage. These compounds support heart health by reducing the risk of chronic diseases and promoting improved blood flow.

- Regular consumption of cacao has been linked to lower blood pressure, contributing to cardiovascular well-being.

### 2. Mood Enhancement and Mental Clarity:

- Cacao contains serotonin precursors, which can elevate mood and alleviate feelings of depression, fostering a sense of well-being.

- Theobromine and a small amount of caffeine within cacao offer a gentle energy boost, enhancing mental alertness without the jitters associated with coffee.

### 3. Essential Minerals:

- Rich in iron, magnesium, and potassium, cacao supports muscle function, energy production, and bone health, making it a holistic addition to a wellness-focused diet.

## Bananas: Nature's Energy and Mood Stabilizer

Bananas are not just a staple fruit worldwide; they are a source of comfort and sustenance, offering a burst of natural sweetness and a host of health benefits.

### 1. Digestive and Heart Health:

- The dietary fiber in bananas, primarily soluble fiber (pectin), supports healthy digestion and regularity. It may also help manage cholesterol levels, promoting cardiovascular health.

- The potassium in bananas aids in regulating blood pressure, maintaining heart function, and balancing bodily fluids.

### 2. Quick, Sustained Energy:

- Bananas contain natural sugars—fructose, glucose, and sucrose—providing a fast yet sustained energy release, ideal for pre- or post-exercise nutrition.

### 3. Brain and Mood Support:

- The high content of vitamin B6 in bananas aids cognitive function and the synthesis of serotonin and dopamine, which are crucial for regulating mood and sleep.

- Antioxidants like dopamine and vitamin C combat free radicals, preserving cellular health.

## Portobello and Cremini Mushrooms: Earthy and Nutritious Allies

Mushrooms, particularly portobello and cremini, bridge the gap between plant and protein sources, enriching meals with texture and nutritional value.

### 1. Nutrient-Dense and Immune-Boosting:

- These mushrooms are packed with protein, fiber, B vitamins (like riboflavin, niacin, and pantothenic acid), and minerals such as selenium and copper, essential for metabolism and immunity.

- The presence of beta-glucans, dietary fibers known to boost immune response, adds to their health-promoting profile.

### 2. Heart and Bone Health:

- Antioxidants like ergothioneine and glutathione help protect the heart by reducing oxidative stress.

- Minerals such as copper and phosphorus play a significant role in maintaining strong bones and healthy nerves.

### 3. Weight and Blood Sugar Management:

- Low in calories and high in fiber, mushrooms support weight management and can help regulate blood sugar levels by moderating carbohydrate absorption.

## Coconut Milk: A Creamy and Nourishing Plant-Based Alternative

Coconut milk, derived from blending coconut flesh with water, is cherished for its rich texture and subtle sweetness. Beyond its culinary appeal, it nurtures the body in meaningful ways.

### 1. Energizing Healthy Fats:

- Rich in medium-chain triglycerides (MCTs), coconut milk offers quick energy while promoting satiety. MCTs are more readily used by the body compared to long-chain fats, making them a favored choice for those seeking sustained energy.

### 2. Immune and Antioxidant Support:

- The lauric acid in coconut milk exhibits antimicrobial and antiviral properties, bolstering the body's defenses.

- Phenolic antioxidants within coconut milk neutralize harmful free radicals, reducing oxidative damage.

### 3. Hydration and Digestive Health:

- Coconut milk is abundant in electrolytes like potassium and sodium and aids in fluid balance and muscle function.

- Its dietary fiber content contributes to healthy digestion and may help regulate blood sugar, making it suitable for diverse nutritional preferences.

## Grass-Fed Butter: A Return to Natural, Nutrient-Dense Nutrition

Grass-fed butter is more than just a kitchen staple – it is a symbol of a return to traditional, whole-food nutrition. Unlike conventional butter, which is typically derived from grain-fed cows, grass-fed butter is sourced from cows that are allowed to graze freely on pastures, resulting in a product that is richer in nutrients and free from many additives.

### *Key Nutrients in Grass-Fed Butter:*

- **Omega-3 Fatty Acids:** Known for their anti-inflammatory properties and critical role in brain and heart health, grass-fed butter contains significantly higher omega-3 fatty acids like alpha-linolenic acid (ALA) than conventional butter.

- **Conjugated Linoleic Acid (CLA):** This unique fatty acid is associated with potential cancer-fighting properties, reduced body fat, and improved immune function. CLA is found in much higher concentrations in grass-fed dairy products.

- **Vitamins A, K2, and E:** Grass-fed butter is a potent source of these fat-soluble vitamins. Vitamin A supports vision and immune function, K2 plays a critical role in bone and cardiovascular health, and vitamin E acts as a powerful antioxidant.

- **Butyrate:** A short-chain fatty acid known for its anti-inflammatory properties.

### *Health Benefits of Grass-Fed Butter:*

- **Heart Health:** With a healthier omega-3 to omega-6 ratio, grass-fed butter may support cardiovascular health by reducing inflammation and supporting healthy blood pressure levels.

- **Enhanced Nutrient Absorption:** Healthy fats aid in the absorption of fat-soluble vitamins, amplifying the nutritional benefits of other foods.

- **Brain Function and Mental Well-being:** The combination of omega-3s, CLA, and butyrate in grass-fed butter is thought to support cognitive function, reduce brain fog, and promote emotional well-being.

## Ghee: An Ancient Elixir of Digestive Health and Longevity

Ghee, a staple of Ayurvedic medicine for centuries, is a form of clarified butter offering various health benefits, particularly for those sensitive to dairy. By removing milk solids, ghee becomes a highly digestible, lactose-free option that retains many of the nutrients found in grass-fed butter.

### Key Nutrients in Ghee:

- **Healthy Saturated Fats:** Ghee is rich in medium-chain fatty acids that are quickly metabolized by the liver, providing a fast source of energy.

- **Conjugated Linoleic Acid (CLA):** Like grass-fed butter, ghee is a potent source of CLA, known for its immune-boosting and potential fat-burning properties.

- **Vitamins A, E, and K2:** These essential vitamins support immune health, bone strength, and cellular repair.

### Health Benefits of Ghee:

- **Lactose and Casein Free:** Ideal for those with dairy sensitivities, as it lacks the milk sugars and proteins that can trigger digestive discomfort.

- **High Smoke Point:** Ghee remains stable at higher temperatures, making it an excellent choice for sautéing and frying without producing harmful free radicals.

- **Digestive Health:** Ghee's butyrate content supports gut health, reducing inflammation and promoting a healthy microbiome.

## Bison Meat: Lean, Nutritious, and Wildly Healthful

Bison meat represents a leaner, more nutrient-dense alternative to conventional beef, reflecting a more natural, less industrialized approach to livestock farming. Bison are typically pasture-raised, making meat free from hormones, antibiotics, and synthetic additives.

### *Key Nutrients in Bison Meat:*

- **Lean Protein:** Bison is lower in fat and calories compared to beef, making it a high-quality source of protein for muscle repair and overall health.

- **Vitamins and Minerals:** Bison is rich in iron, zinc, vitamin B12, selenium, and niacin – nutrients essential for energy production, immune function, and cognitive health.

- **Omega-3 Fatty Acids:** While not as high as fish, bison meat offers a more balanced omega-3 to omega-6 ratio compared to conventional meats, promoting heart health and reducing inflammation.

### *Health Benefits of Bison Meat:*

- **Heart Health:** The lean nature and favorable fatty acid profile of bison make it a heart-friendly choice.

- **Reduced Inflammation:** Lower omega-6 levels help reduce chronic inflammation, a key factor in many modern health issues.

- **Sustainable Nutrition:** Bison farming often aligns with regenerative agricultural practices, supporting environmental health and biodiversity.

## Nourishing Grains and Plant-Based Options

- **Ezekiel Bread:** Made from sprouted whole grains and legumes, this bread offers a complete amino acid profile, supporting muscle repair and energy levels while being easier to digest due to the breakdown of antinutrients during sprouting.

- **Bamboo Tea:** High in silica, bamboo tea promotes bone, skin, and hair health, adding a unique mineral boost to your diet.

## Medjool Dates and Blackstrap Molasses

## Medjool Dates:

## Constituents:

- **Natural Sugars** (Fructose and Glucose): Medjool dates are naturally rich in sugars, providing a quick and sustained energy boost, making them a popular choice for athletes and those seeking natural energy sources.

- **Dietary Fiber:** Dates contain both soluble and insoluble fiber, supporting healthy digestion, promoting regular bowel movements, and helping regulate blood sugar levels by slowing sugar absorption.

- **Vitamins and Minerals:** Dates are packed with essential nutrients, including potassium, magnesium, calcium, and vitamin B6, which are vital for heart health, bone strength, and overall cellular function.

## Health Benefits:

- **Digestive Health:** High fiber content in dates supports a healthy digestive system, helps prevent constipation, and promotes regular bowel movements.

- **Heart Health:** Rich in potassium and magnesium, dates help regulate blood pressure, support heart function, and reduce the risk of stroke.

- **Natural Energy Boost:** Dates provide a rapid energy boost due to their natural sugar content, making them ideal for pre-workout fuel.

- **Bone Health:** The minerals in dates, including calcium and magnesium, support bone density and help prevent osteoporosis.

- **Antioxidant Properties:** Dates contain polyphenols and flavonoids, powerful antioxidants that protect cells from oxidative damage and reduce inflammation.

**Blackstrap Molasses:**

**Constituents:**

- **Iron:** Blackstrap molasses is a highly concentrated source of iron, essential for oxygen transport in the blood and preventing iron-deficiency anemia.

- **Calcium and Magnesium:** These minerals are critical for bone health, muscle function, and nerve signaling.

- **Potassium:** Important for heart health, blood pressure regulation, and muscle function.

- **B Vitamins:** Includes B6, niacin, riboflavin, and pantothenic acid, supporting energy metabolism, nerve function, and overall cellular health.

**Health Benefits:**

- **Iron Boost:** Blackstrap molasses is a valuable source of iron, particularly beneficial for those with anemia or increased iron needs, such as pregnant women.

- **Bone Health:** High levels of calcium and magnesium support bone density and help prevent osteoporosis.

- **Heart Health:** Potassium content supports cardiovascular health by helping regulate blood pressure and maintaining heart rhythm.

- **Energy and Muscle Function:** The rich mineral profile supports energy production, muscle function, and overall metabolic health.

- **Menstrual Health:** The iron content in blackstrap molasses can help alleviate symptoms of menstrual discomfort and fatigue.

**How They Work Together:** Both Medjool dates and blackstrap molasses provide natural, nutrient-dense sources of energy, fiber, and essential minerals. Their combination can support digestive health, bone strength, and overall vitality, making them ideal for those seeking natural, whole-food-based energy sources.

However, due to their high natural sugar content, they should be consumed in moderation, and it's advisable to consult with a healthcare professional if you have specific health conditions.

**Blueberries and Strawberries:**

**Blueberries:**

**Constituents:**

- **Antioxidants:** Blueberries are rich in anthocyanins, which give them their deep blue color and potent antioxidant properties.

- **Vitamins and Minerals:** They provide significant amounts of vitamins C and K, as well as manganese, supporting immune function, bone health, and overall vitality.

- **Dietary Fiber:** Blueberries are a great source of dietary fiber, supporting digestive health and helping regulate blood sugar levels.

**Health Benefits:**

- **Antioxidant Powerhouse:** Blueberries are among the highest antioxidant-rich fruits, protecting cells from oxidative stress and potentially reducing the risk of chronic diseases like heart disease and cancer.

- **Brain Health:** Research suggests that the antioxidants in blueberries may improve cognitive function, enhance memory, and delay brain aging.

- **Heart Health:** Regular consumption of blueberries may lower blood pressure, reduce LDL cholesterol, and support overall cardiovascular health.

- **Anti-Inflammatory Properties:** The antioxidants and phytochemicals in blueberries help reduce inflammation, a key factor in many chronic diseases.

- Blood Sugar Regulation: Blueberries may improve insulin sensitivity and support healthy blood sugar levels, making them beneficial for individuals with diabetes.

## Strawberries:

## Constituents:

- **Vitamins and Minerals:** Strawberries are an excellent source of vitamin C, folate, potassium, and manganese, supporting immune function, heart health, and overall well-being.

- **Antioxidants:** Strawberries contain anthocyanins, ellagic acid, and quercetin, powerful antioxidants that protect against oxidative stress and inflammation.

- **Dietary Fiber:** Strawberries provide good dietary fiber, supporting digestion and promoting a sense of fullness.

**Health Benefits:**

- **Antioxidant and Anti-Inflammatory Properties:** Strawberries' rich antioxidant profile helps reduce oxidative stress, combat inflammation, and potentially lower the risk of chronic diseases.

- **Heart Health:** Regular consumption of strawberries can help lower blood pressure, reduce LDL cholesterol, and improve overall heart health.

- **Immune Support:** High vitamin C content boosts the immune system, helping the body fend off infections and recover from illness.

- **Skin Health:** Antioxidants in strawberries promote healthy, youthful skin by reducing oxidative damage and supporting collagen production.

- **Blood Sugar Regulation:** With a low glycemic index, strawberries can help regulate blood sugar levels, making them a healthy choice for those managing diabetes.

**How They Work Together:** Blueberries and strawberries are nutrient-dense, antioxidant-rich fruits that support overall health. Their combination provides a powerful mix of vitamins, minerals, and fiber, promoting heart, brain, and immune health while helping regulate blood sugar levels. Including these berries in a balanced diet can enhance overall well-being, but it's essential to consume them as part of a varied diet for maximum benefit.

## Methylsulfonylmethane (MSM)

### *Overview*

Methylsulfonylmethane, commonly known as MSM, is a sulfur-containing compound often consumed as a dietary supplement, typically in powder form. It is valued for its potential health benefits, particularly related to sulfur and methyl group metabolism.

### *Key Constituents*

MSM is a naturally occurring compound found in plants, animals, and humans. It consists of carbon, hydrogen, oxygen, and sulfur atoms. The sulfur component makes MSM a rich source of bioavailable sulfur, which is crucial for maintaining healthy bodily functions.

### *Health Benefits*

- **Joint Health:**

  MSM supports joint health by providing bioavailable sulfur, essential for collagen formation. Collagen is a key structural protein in connective tissues, cartilage, and tendons.

- **Pain and Inflammation Management:**

  MSM has been studied for its anti-inflammatory properties, which may help alleviate pain and discomfort, particularly in conditions like osteoarthritis and muscle soreness.

- **Skin Health:**

  Sulfur plays a vital role in collagen synthesis, promoting skin elasticity and reducing signs of aging. MSM may help maintain healthy, vibrant skin.

- **Hair and Nail Health:**

  As a fundamental component of keratin, sulfur derived from MSM may enhance hair strength and nail health.

- **Allergy Relief:**

  Some studies suggest MSM may exhibit antihistamine properties, potentially reducing symptoms like sneezing, itching, and congestion.

- **Exercise Recovery:**

  MSM may reduce muscle damage and oxidative stress after intense physical activity, aiding in quicker recovery.

- **Detoxification:**

  Sulfur from MSM supports the body's detoxification pathways, including the synthesis of glutathione, an antioxidant vital for eliminating toxins.

### *How MSM Works*

MSM serves as a source of organic sulfur, essential for synthesizing amino acids, enzymes, and other critical molecules. It also supports methylation, a biochemical process vital for DNA synthesis, neurotransmitter production, and detoxification. Incorporating MSM into the diet may support joint, skin, and overall health, but consulting a healthcare provider before use is recommended.

**Coconuts and Coconut Water**

*Key Constituents*

- **Medium-Chain Triglycerides (MCTs):**

  These fats are metabolized differently, providing a quick energy source.

- **Electrolytes:**

  Coconut water contains potassium, sodium, magnesium, and calcium, making it an excellent natural hydration drink.

- **Antioxidants:**

  Both coconut flesh and water contain antioxidants that protect cells from oxidative stress.

**Vitamins and Minerals:**

Includes vitamin C, B vitamins, iron, and phosphorus, which are essential for overall health.

*Health Benefits*

- **Hydration:**

  Due to its high electrolyte content, coconut water is ideal for rehydration, especially after physical exertion.

- **Heart Health:**

  MCTs may help boost HDL (good cholesterol) levels, potentially supporting cardiovascular health.

- **Digestive Health:**

  The dietary fiber in coconuts supports gut health and regular bowel movements.

- **Immune Support:**

  Rich in vitamins and antioxidants, coconuts may enhance the immune response.

- **Skin and Hair Care:**

  Coconut oil's moisturizing properties make it beneficial for maintaining healthy skin and hair.

- **Weight Management:**

  MCTs may promote satiety and support metabolism.

### *How They Work*

Coconut components, particularly MCTs, provide a quick energy boost. The high electrolyte content in coconut water aids in maintaining fluid balance. Additionally, the antioxidants combat free radicals, while dietary fiber promotes gut health.

### Arugula

### *Key Constituents*

- **Vitamins and Minerals:**

  Rich in vitamins A, C, K, folate, calcium, potassium, and iron.

- **Antioxidants:**

  Contains compounds like vitamin C that help reduce oxidative damage.

- **Phytochemicals:**

  Includes glucosinolates, which may offer cancer-protective effects.

- **Nitrates:**

  These compounds may improve blood flow and enhance exercise performance.

### *Health Benefits*

- **Bone Health:**

  High vitamin K content supports bone density and may reduce osteoporosis risk.

- **Heart Health:**

  Nitrates can help lower blood pressure, while antioxidants support cardiovascular function.

- **Anti-Inflammatory:**

  The phytochemicals may reduce inflammation and the risk of chronic diseases.

- **Digestive Health:**

  Fiber in arugula aids digestion and promotes gut health.

- **Immune Support:**

  Rich in vitamin C, arugula bolsters the body's natural defenses.

### *How It Works*

Arugula's vitamins and antioxidants support metabolic processes and help reduce inflammation. The presence of dietary nitrates may enhance blood circulation, contributing to cardiovascular health.

**Pomegranates and Avocados**

*Pomegranates*

- **Antioxidants:**

  Contains punicalagins and anthocyanins, which help reduce oxidative stress.

- **Vitamins and Minerals:**

  Rich in vitamin C, K, potassium, and folate.

- **Fiber:**

  Aids in digestion and supports gut health.

*Health Benefits*

- **Heart Health:**

  Antioxidants may lower blood pressure and reduce cholesterol.

- **Anti-Inflammatory:**

  Potentially decreases the risk of chronic conditions.

- **Digestive Health:**

  Fiber helps regulate bowel movements.

*Avocados*

- **Healthy Fats:**

  High in monounsaturated fats like oleic acid, which are beneficial for heart health.

- **Vitamins and Minerals:**

  Contains vitamins C, E, K, B vitamins, and potassium.

- **Fiber:**

Supports digestive health and satiety.

### *Health Benefits*

- **Heart Health:**

May lower LDL cholesterol and support vascular function.

- **Weight Management:**

High fiber and healthy fats aid in controlling appetite.

- **Blood Sugar Control:**

Low glycemic index makes it suitable for diabetics.

**Hemp Seed Oil**

*Key Constituents*

- **Essential Fatty Acids:**

  Rich in omega-3 (ALA) and omega-6 (LA), crucial for cardiovascular and cognitive health.

- **Gamma-Linolenic Acid (GLA):**

  Supports anti-inflammatory responses and hormonal balance.

- **Antioxidants:**

  Contains vitamin E to combat oxidative stress.

- **Phytosterols:**

  May help reduce LDL cholesterol levels.

*Health Benefits*

- **Heart Health:**

  Balances omega-3 and omega-6 intake, promoting cardiovascular well-being.

- **Skin Health:**

  GLA can alleviate conditions like eczema.

- **Anti-Inflammatory:**

  Supports immune health and may reduce joint pain.

## Final Thoughts: Choosing Foods That Sustain Life

In a society facing rising rates of chronic illness, the foods we choose carry deep emotional and physiological weight. Bell peppers, watermelon, kiwi, salmon, and sardines offer more than calories—they offer **capacity**. Capacity for healing, resilience, mental clarity, and joy. They provide the biochemical foundations that keep us upright and thriving.

When we nourish ourselves with intention—drawing from nature's most vibrant offerings—we honor the intelligence of the body and the Earth alike. It is not just a matter of nutrition; it is a matter of reverence.

Including these nutrient-rich ingredients in your diet can significantly contribute to overall health and well-being. However, as with any dietary supplement or health food, consulting a healthcare professional is recommended to ensure safety and efficacy.

# NURTURING HEALTH THROUGH LOW-IMPACT EXERCISE

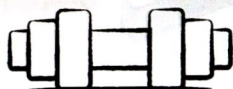

Crystal had always been an avid enthusiast of high-impact aerobics and jogging. It was her escape, her sanctuary, and her favorite way to maintain her cardiovascular health. But her life took a turn when she was diagnosed with Paget's disease; the pain that accompanied this condition made her cherished high-impact exercises an agonizing challenge. She was faced with a difficult decision - surrender to her limitations or find an alternative that would allow her to maintain her fitness while accommodating her condition.

Determined to keep her health a priority despite the hurdles, Crystal embarked on a journey to discover exercises that were gentle on her joints yet effective in promoting cardiovascular health and muscle toning. She incorporated swimming and walking on the treadmill into her fitness routine.

## The Power of Swimming:

## Low-Impact, High-Resistance Training

Swimming is a remarkable exercise that perfectly balances low-impact movement and high-resistance training. When you submerge yourself in a refreshing pool, you will experience the unique resistance provided by the water, making every stroke and kick a powerful workout for your muscles.

The water's resistance acts as a natural weight, making each movement a strength-building exercise. As you extend your arms and pull yourself through the water, the resistance will challenge your biceps, triceps, and pectoral muscles. Similarly, the powerful leg kicks will engage your quadriceps, hamstrings, and calf muscles. It is a full-body strength training session, but in a gentle and supportive environment.

The beauty of water is that it provides multi-directional resistance, forcing muscles to work against the water's pressure from all angles. This helps tone and strengthen the muscles in a balanced way, contributing to a leaner and more defined physique. Despite the muscle engagement, the low-impact nature of swimming ensures that the stress on the joints and bones is minimal, making it ideal for individuals like Crystal who needed to be cautious of high-impact activities due to Paget's disease.

As you glide through the water, you will feel your heart rate gradually increase, a testament to the incredible cardiovascular benefits of swimming. Swimming is an exceptional aerobic exercise that efficiently elevates the heart rate, enhancing cardiovascular endurance and improving overall heart health.

During swimming, the body continuously moves against the water's resistance, requiring the heart to pump more oxygenated blood to the muscles. This heightened oxygen demand stimulates the heart, improving its strength and efficiency. Over time, regular swimming sessions led to a lowered resting heart rate, a key indicator of an efficient cardiovascular system.

Swimming is also a great way to improve lung capacity and function. The rhythmic breathing pattern while swimming, inhaling as the head is turned to the side and exhaling underwater, enhances lung efficiency and capacity. This improved respiratory function allows the body to utilize oxygen more effectively during exercise and daily activities.

Moreover, the repetitive nature of swimming, combined with the engagement of major muscle groups, ensures a sustained increase in heart rate throughout the workout. This continuous cardiovascular activity helps burn calories and maintain a healthy weight, reducing the risk of chronic diseases like obesity, diabetes, and hypertension.

Crystal soon realized that swimming was not just a recreational activity; it was her lifeline to maintaining optimal cardiovascular health in a manner that was gentle and accommodating to her condition. It became an exercise deeply woven into her routine, providing her with physical strength and the peace and solace that comes with being in the water.

**Walking**

**A Low-Impact Exercise with High-Impact Benefits**

Walking is often underestimated as a form of exercise, but its benefits are substantial and can be a cornerstone of a healthy, low-impact fitness routine. For individuals like Crystal, who needed to be mindful of the strain on her joints, walking was a valuable exercise that provided an effective workout without putting excessive stress on the body.

1. **Low-Impact on Joints and Bones:** Walking is a low-impact exercise, making it gentle on the joints and bones. The natural motion of walking allows for fluid movement in the joints without the jarring impact that high-impact exercises can have. For someone whose bones or joints are weakened by Paget's disease or arthritis, this is crucial. It can help maintain mobility, improve bone density, and reduce the risk of fractures or further damage.

2. **Muscle Toning and Strength:** Contrary to popular belief, walking is an excellent way to tone and strengthen muscles. While it might not have the same intensity as weightlifting or resistance training, walking engages various muscle groups throughout the body. The legs, glutes, core, and even the arms are utilized during the walking motion. The consistent engagement of these muscles helps in toning and improving muscle strength over time.

3. **Cardiovascular Benefits:** Walking is a powerful aerobic exercise that significantly benefits cardiovascular health. It raises the heart rate and increases circulation, promoting improved cardiovascular endurance. As Crystal would walk

briskly, her heart would pump more blood and oxygen to her muscles, improving their efficiency and endurance. This cardiovascular workout reduced the risk of heart disease, stroke, and high blood pressure.

4. **Weight Management and Calorie Burning:** Regular walking, especially at a brisk pace, can aid in weight management and calorie burning. It's an effective way to burn calories, contributing to weight loss or weight maintenance.

   When combined with a balanced diet, regular walking can help you manage weight, which is crucial for overall health and managing the effects of Paget's disease.

5. **Mental Health and Stress Reduction:** Walking isn't just beneficial for the body; it's good for the mind. It helps reduce stress and anxiety and promotes mental well-being. The rhythmic movement and being in nature (if walking outdoors) can have a calming effect on the mind, improving mood and reducing symptoms of depression.

Crystal found walking to be a sanctuary—a simple yet powerful exercise that allowed her to maintain her health, both physically and mentally. It became her daily ritual, a time to reflect, rejuvenate, and focus on her well-being. Despite its seemingly simple nature, walking played a significant role in her journey towards a healthier and more fulfilling life, proving that sometimes the most effective solutions are the ones grounded in simplicity.

# EMBRACING THE FASTING LIFESTYLE

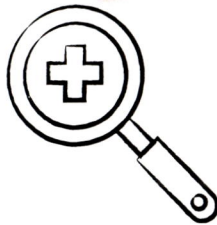

In our pursuit of a healthier and more balanced lifestyle, we embarked on a journey to embrace fasting as a way to optimize our health and well-being. Our fasting adventure began with a gradual adjustment of the time we consumed our first meal, commonly known as breakfast.

Initially, we were accustomed to having our first meal shortly after waking up, around 8 am. However, we desired to experiment with a fasting routine, extending the period between our last meal of the previous day and our first meal of the current day. The objective was to benefit from the metabolic advantages that fasting can offer.

We decided to shift our breakfast time by one hour each week until we reached a target of 1 pm. This allowed our bodies to adapt gradually to the extended fasting window, making the transition smooth and sustainable.

## Understanding Fasting and Its Effects

**Meal Fasting:** Meal fasting, or intermittent fasting, is an eating pattern that involves cycling between periods of eating and fasting. It doesn't specify which foods you should eat but instead focuses on when you should eat. This practice allows the body to utilize stored energy, promoting fat burning and other health benefits.

As we pushed our breakfast time further into the day, we effectively extended our fasting window. This approach promoted autophagy, the body's process of cleaning out damaged cells and regenerating new ones. Autophagy has various health benefits, including reduced inflammation and a lower risk of chronic diseases.

**Ketosis and Ketones:** During fasting, especially in a prolonged fasting state, the body depletes its glycogen reserves, shifting to an alternative fuel source called ketones. Ketones are small fuel molecules produced by the liver from fatty acids. This metabolic state is known as ketosis.

Ketosis provides the body and brain with a highly efficient and sustainable energy source. When in ketosis, the body burns fat for fuel, aiding in weight loss and body fat reduction. Ketones have also been linked to improved mental clarity and focus, making fasting an appealing option for increased productivity.

**The Benefits of Fasting**

1. **Weight Management:** Fasting can assist in weight management by reducing calorie intake and promoting fat loss. The shift to utilizing stored fat for energy during fasting contributes to weight loss, making it an effective tool for those seeking to manage their weight.

2. **Improved Insulin Sensitivity:** Fasting enhances insulin sensitivity, enabling better blood sugar control. This is crucial in preventing insulin resistance, a precursor to type 2 diabetes. By reducing the frequency of meals, fasting allows the body to regulate insulin levels more effectively.

3. **Cellular Repair and Longevity:** Autophagy, stimulated during fasting, is a process that facilitates the repair and recycling of damaged cells. This cellular rejuvenation promotes longevity and helps prevent various age-related diseases.

4. **Cognitive Benefits:** Ketones, the byproduct of fasting-induced ketosis, are known to be a highly efficient brain fuel. Fasting can lead to improved cognitive function, focus, and mental clarity. It may also reduce the risk of neurodegenerative disorders.

As we gradually adjusted our eating schedule and embraced fasting, we reaped the rewards of improved health and vitality. The transformative power of fasting inspired us to continue exploring this lifestyle, appreciating the profound impact it can have on our overall well-being.

# BREAKING OUR FAST - THE NOURISHING SHAKE

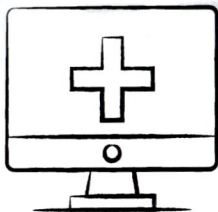

The clock struck 1 PM, signaling the end of our fasting period. It was a moment we had eagerly awaited, the moment to break our fast and fuel our bodies after hours of abstaining from food. But breaking the fast wasn't about indulging in a hearty meal; it was about nourishing our bodies wisely with a carefully crafted protein shake.

## Our Philosophy of the Shake

In our journey toward a healthier lifestyle, we adopted intermittent fasting to promote better overall well-being. Intermittent fasting provided numerous benefits, ranging from weight management to improved metabolic health. Our fasting window typically lasted from the previous evening until 1 PM the following day, totaling roughly 19 hours without food.

Breaking this fast was a crucial moment in our daily routine. We had chosen a protein shake as our first post-fast meal, and for good reason. The philosophy behind starting the day with a protein shake was rooted in providing our bodies with a quick and easily digestible source of essential nutrients, without burdening our digestive system with a heavy meal.

Our chosen shake was carefully crafted to include a balance of high-quality protein, healthy fats, vitamins, and minerals. It contained 2-3 bananas, 4- 5 cups of coconut milk, 2 tablespoons of cacao powder, 1 tablespoon of blackstrap molasses, 2 medjool dates, $\frac{1}{2}$ tablespoon of hemp seed oil, 1 tablespoon of nutritional yeast, $\frac{1}{2}$ teaspoon of Ceylon cinnamon, $\frac{1}{2}$ teaspoon of Ashwagandha, and two tablespoons of pea protein powder.

**Here are some of the benefits we reaped from consuming this nutritious shake:**

- **Rapid Nutrient Absorption**: The liquid form of a shake allowed for faster digestion and absorption of nutrients. After a fast, our bodies were primed to efficiently absorb essential nutrients, making a protein shake an ideal choice.

- **Protein for Muscle Recovery and Growth**: Protein is essential for repairing and building muscle tissue. By starting our day with a protein-rich shake, we ensured our muscles received the necessary amino acids to recover and grow, especially after a workout.

- **Steady Energy Release**: The combination of protein, healthy fats, and carbohydrates in the shake provided a balanced and sustained release of energy throughout the day. This steadiness in energy levels helped us remain focused and productive.

- **Metabolic Boost**: Protein has a higher thermic effect compared to fats and carbohydrates, meaning it requires more energy to digest. Consuming a protein-rich shake kick-started our metabolism, encouraging efficient calorie burning.

- **Appetite Control**: Protein is well-known for its ability to promote feelings of fullness and satiety. Starting our day with a protein shake helped control our appetite, reducing the likelihood of overeating later in the day.

**The Digestive Advantage**

One of the significant advantages of consuming a protein shake as the first meal after fasting was the minimal impact on the digestive system. After a period of fasting, the digestive tract is in a state of rest, making it more sensitive to the type and quantity of food consumed.

A well-blended, easily digestible shake allowed our bodies to absorb essential nutrients efficiently without overwhelming our digestive system. The liquid form of the shake required less effort from the digestive organs, allowing the body to direct its energy toward absorbing nutrients and initiating the metabolic processes crucial for the day ahead.

As we sipped on our carefully prepared protein shake, we were reminded of the conscious choices we made to prioritize Crystal's health. Breaking our fast with this nourishing shake was not just a dietary decision; it was a step toward ensuring her body received the optimal nutrients in a manner that supported her wellness journey.

With each sip, she not only fueled her body for the day ahead but also for the years to come, confident in the positive impact this mindful choice would have on her overall health and well-being.

In 2023, Crystal's alkaline phosphatase level has decreased from the initially high and abnormal value of 532 to a normal range of 81, still slightly elevated but within acceptable norms.

As of 2024, Crystal's alkaline phosphatase continues to drop. Now at a level of 76.

Crystal's metabolic disorder was reversed. She no longer suffers from the pain of Paget's Disease of the bone or arthritis.

# CONCLUSION

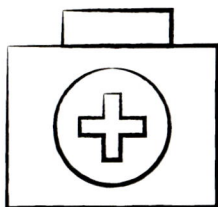

As we bring this book to a close, we can't help but reflect on how little we understood about the profound connection between our diets and health when we first embarked on this journey in 2012. At that time, conversations around food and wellness were scarce, and the importance of eating organic, non-GMO foods wasn't the household concept it has become today. Social media platforms were still in their infancy as tools for spreading awareness about nutrition, and most of us were following habits passed down or driven by convenience.

But as we began to experiment with changing our eating habits, the results spoke for themselves—loudly and clearly. What started as a slight adjustment to what we put on our plates grew into a transformative lifestyle shift. Over time, we watched in amazement as Crystal's health improved dramatically. Not only did her symptoms subside, but she also started to defy the health challenges so often deemed inevitable by society.

Now, at 60 years young, Crystal is a living testament to the power of dietary change. A beautiful African American woman, she stands strong and vibrant, free from the chronic conditions that disproportionately affect our African American community, such as diabetes, high blood pressure, high cholesterol, arthritis, or even the debilitating effects of Paget's disease. The only explanation? A simple yet profound commitment to eating differently.

This journey taught us that it's never too late to reclaim control of your health. Small, deliberate changes in your diet can lead to profound improvements in your well-being.

You don't need to wait for a crisis to start—it's as simple as prioritizing whole, natural, and nourishing foods today.

We hope Crystal's story has inspired you as much as it has inspired us. Our mission in sharing this journey is to empower you to take the reins of your health and realize that you have the ability to feel better, live stronger, and thrive in ways you may not have thought possible.

The old saying "you are what you eat" is more than a catchy phrase; it's a truth we've come to live by. As we close this book, we encourage you to open a new chapter in your life—a chapter that prioritizes self-care, mindful choices, and the belief that your health is worth every ounce of effort you put into it.

Remember, the journey to wellness begins with one bite, one step, and one decision at a time.

Here's to your health, your journey, and your transformation.

With Loving Intentions,

*James and Crystal Bass*

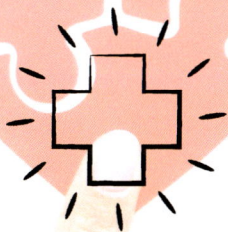
RECEIPTS

Name: Crystal ██████████ | ████ | ██████ | PCP ███████ MD | Legal Name: Crystal ████████ Bass

## ALKALINE PHOS
Collected on August 29, 2012 10:35

Lab tests - Blood

Results

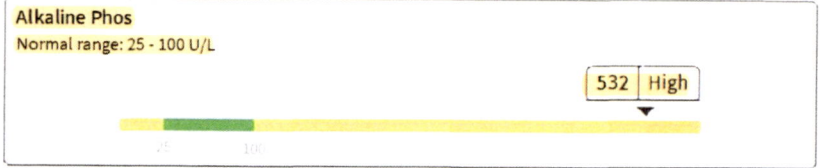

**Alkaline Phos**
Normal range: 25 - 100 U/L

532 | High

# CT HEAD WO CONTRAST

Collected on October 31, 2013 19 46

## Results  New

### Impression

IMPRESSION:
1. No acute intracranial pathology.
2. Incidental note of a mottled heterogeneous skull noted within the diploic space, patient had bone scan of 12/10/12 which indicated uptake throughout the skull characteristic of Padgett's disease however patient has also had history of uterine cancer. Findings can be associated with metabolic disorders, metastatic disease. Correlate clinically.

Narrative

NONCONTRAST HEAD CT 10/31/13
INDICATION:
Pain, trauma.
TECHNIQUE:
5 mm non-enhanced axial images through the brain. Multiplanar reformations obtained. The DLP for this procedure was 995 mGy-cm.
FINDINGS:
Sulci and ventricles are normal for age. No acute intracranial hemorrhage, mass, nor abnormal extraaxial fluid collections. Basal cisterns are preserved. No inferior cerebellar tonsillar ectopia. Sella region within normal limits. Orbits unremarkable. Nasopharyngeal soft tissues unremarkable. Visualized paranasal sinuses and mastoid air cells clear. No acute fractures identified. There is however mottled appearance to the diploic space of the skull with increased sclerosis noted diffusely through the diploic space. No fracture is identified.
6997436

# CT HEAD WO CONTRAST

2014 07 31

## Results  New

### Impression

IMPRESSION:
1. No evidence of intracranial hemorrhage or contusion.
2. Abnormal calvarial mineralization pattern consistent with known history of Paget disease.

### Narrative

CT HEAD WITHOUT CONTRAST 08/24/14 0733 HOURS
HISTORY:
Altered neurologic status. Syncope. Status post fall. Known history of Paget disease.
TECHNIQUE:
5 mm non-enhanced axial images through the brain. Multiplanar reformations obtained.
COMPARISON:
10/31/13.
FINDINGS:
A right frontal scalp focal contusion is visualized. No underlying calvarial fracture. The calvarium is abnormally thickened and has a coarsened mineralization pattern consistent with the known history of Paget disease. No other interval change compared to 10/31/13. No focus of abnormal intracranial attenuation suspicious for hemorrhage or contusion. No midline shift or basilar cistern effacement. The ventricles are non-dilated.
The paranasal sinuses and mastoid air cells remain clear.
7527139

Test Details

# LIVER PANEL

Collected on January 17, 2023 07 13

## Lab tests - Blood (Plasma)

Results

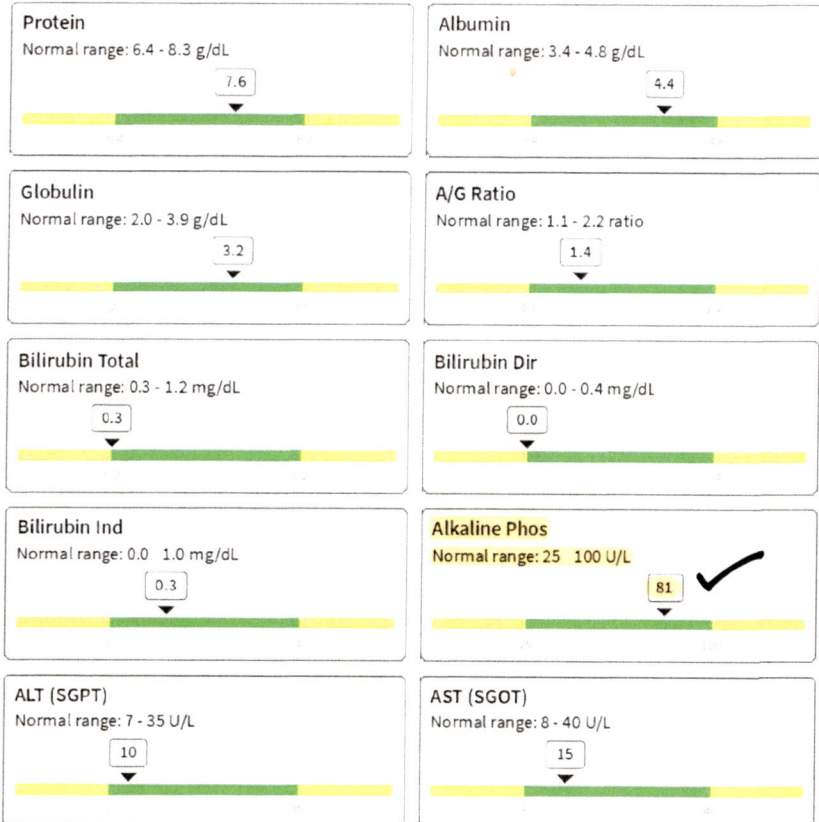

**Protein**
Normal range: 6.4 - 8.3 g/dL

7.6

**Albumin**
Normal range: 3.4 - 4.8 g/dL

4.4

**Globulin**
Normal range: 2.0 - 3.9 g/dL

3.2

**A/G Ratio**
Normal range: 1.1 - 2.2 ratio

1.4

**Bilirubin Total**
Normal range: 0.3 - 1.2 mg/dL

0.3

**Bilirubin Dir**
Normal range: 0.0 - 0.4 mg/dL

0.0

**Bilirubin Ind**
Normal range: 0.0   1.0 mg/dL

0.3

**Alkaline Phos**
Normal range: 25   100 U/L

81 ✓

**ALT (SGPT)**
Normal range: 7 - 35 U/L

10

**AST (SGOT)**
Normal range: 8 - 40 U/L

15

**CARBON DIOXIDE**

Reference Range: 20-32 mmol/L

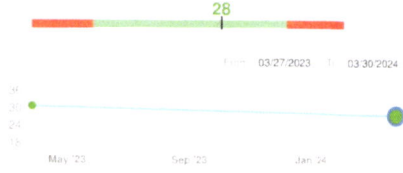

28

From 03/27/2023  To 03/30/2024

May '23          Sep '23          Jan '24

**CALCIUM**

Reference Range: 8.6-10.4 mg/dL

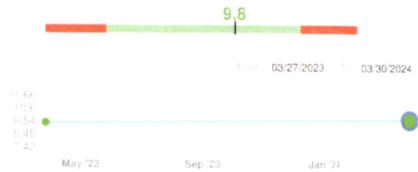

9.8

From 03/27/2023  To 03/30/2024

May '23          Sep '23          Jan '24

**PROTEIN, TOTAL**

Reference Range: 6.1-8.1 g/dL

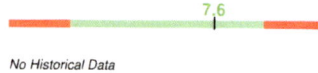

7.6

*No Historical Data*

**ALBUMIN**

Reference Range: 3.6-5.1 g/dL

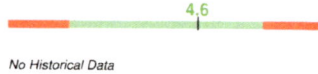

4.6

*No Historical Data*

**GLOBULIN**

Reference Range: 1.9-3.7 g/dL (calc)

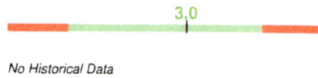

3.0

*No Historical Data*

**ALBUMIN/GLOBULIN RATIO**

Reference Range: 1.0-2.5 (calc)

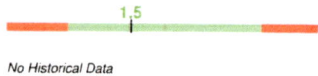

1.5

*No Historical Data*

**BILIRUBIN, TOTAL**

Reference Range: 0.2-1.2 mg/dL

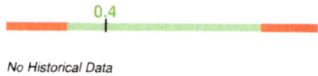

0.4

*No Historical Data*

**ALKALINE PHOSPHATASE**

Reference Range: 37-153 U/L

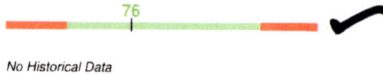

76

*No Historical Data*

**AST**

Reference Range: 10-35 U/L

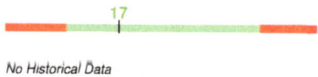

17

*No Historical Data*

**ALT**

Reference Range: 6-29 U/L

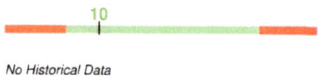

10

*No Historical Data*

www.ingramcontent.com/pod-product-compliance
Lightning Source LLC
Chambersburg PA
CBRC101141030426
42335CB00007B/201